Thyroid Healing: How to Heal Hyperthyroidism, Hashimoto's, Graves', Insomnia, Nodules, & Epstein Barr

By Jahn Novak

Copyright 2018
Third Edition, License Notes

Copyright Info:

Legal Info:

This author and or rights owner(s) make no claims, promises, or guarantees in regards to the accuracy, completeness, or adequacy of the contents of this book, and expressly disclaims liability for errors and omissions in the contents within. This product is for reference use only. Please consult a professional before taking action on any of the contents found within.

Preface

We want to take a moment to say thank you for purchasing our guide online. HiddenStuff Entertainment remains one of the top app and eBook publishers online. It is our commitment to bring you the most important information to enrich your life.

We sincerely hope that you find this guide useful and beneficial in your quest for betterment. We want to provide readers with knowledge and build their skills to perform at the highest levels within their topics of interest. This in turn contributes to a positive and more enjoyable experience. After all, it is our belief that things in life are to be enjoyed as much as they possibly can be.

If you are in need of additional support or resources in regards to this guide, please feel free to visit our webpage at Hiddenstuffentertainment.com

Contents

Introduction

Are you having thyroid problems? If your thyroid isn't functioning the way that it ought to, such can lead to problems such as being stressed out, unhappy and unhealthy. There are lots of functions that your thyroid performs. These could be ensuring that your metabolism is regulated, not making you gain weight unnecessarily, also making your mood to be balanced. It can also help in ensuring that your sleep is smooth through proper digestion. This is the reason why if it isn't working effectively; lots of things will go wrong in your life.

The unfortunate aspect is that thyroid disease seems to be spreading more than ever before. Also, there are lots of those suffering from this problem who haven't been diagnosed.

Whenever you are suspecting to be suffering from thyroid problem, ensure to seek the help of a holistic practitioner in order to carry out all the necessary lab tests. Working alongside a practitioner will help you identify the major cause of your thyroid problem. Once such causes aren't identified, the problem will not be tackled.

Finding An Experienced Holistic Practitioner

Just as said, this problem will not be tackled unless you its primary cause is identified. With an experienced holistic practitioner, this problem can be identified. Also, the most ideal solution based on your system will be recommended.

GI Pathogen Test Should Be Run by Your Practitioner

It is a stool test which is meant at identifying or spotting parasites. Ensure that your intestinal tract doesn't have any parasite infection. Those who test positive to thyroid antibodies always suffer from parasite infection. For the result to be very accurate, your holistic practitioner will need to run the test for about 4 days.

Avoiding Soy

Your thyroid gland can be damaged by soy. This is those important nutrients which will enable the thyroid to function very well will be blocked. Labels should be carefully checked since soybeans oil is being used in most of the packaged products in the market today.

Diet

Staying Away From Gluten

Gluten in US has been discovered to highly acid and inflammatory. It is a major reason why thyroid malfunctions. Gluten leads to autoimmune response in people. Also, it has been discovered to be a major reason why people experience Hashimoto's thyroiditis which is an autoimmune thyroid condition that is common. Gluten can also lead to autoimmune antibody production most especially in people who have TPO levels that are elevated.

Using Coconut Oil

The conversion of T3 to T4 isn't interrupted by coconut oil the way that lots of cooking oils usually do. It will ensure that your metabolism is increased and assist you in losing weight.

Also, it can support GI as well as immune health. These are important for your thyroid to function properly. In place of your baking and cooking oils, you can make use of coconut oil. Also, ensure to take virgin coconut oil (a table spoon) daily. You can also include it in your diet.

All vegetables containing goitrogens should be cooked once you are having hypothyroidism

Thyroid hormone production can be blocked by goitrogens. There are vegetables you should cook once you are trying to tackle thyroid issues. These could be watercress, rutabaga, bok choy, kale, cabbages, brussels sprouts, cauliflower and broccoli.

Peanut butter and peanuts should be avoided

Seaweed as well as other sea vegetables should be eaten

These could be in the form of wakame, kombu and nori. They contain high amount of iodine and also have other wonderful nutritional benefits.

Drinking of bone broth

Bone broth should be taken on daily basis. This should be from pasture raised animals which are healthy. It can help in healing and sealing of the gut lining and also ensures that the immune system is strengthened. These are very important for a healthy thyroid. A cup of bone broth should be taken every day. Just add sea salt (a pinch) and also kelp flakes. This will help to make the thyroid healthy.

Removing Stress and Detox

Thyroid issues can be triggered by stress. Lots of Americans undergo too much stress on a daily basis. This could be as a result of environmental toxins, food toxin, and stress of life. When stress chemicals such as cortisol and adrenalin are being supplied constantly, such can lead to inferring with thyroid hormones thereby causing thyroid disease.

Ensure to de – stress and detox the body regularly. I will suggest Epsom salt baths since they have helped me achieved great results in the past.

Going Natural

The world today is fully of too many chemicals which our systems take in through one means or the other. The air we breathe every day is toxic, food is toxic and we have got beauty related products which are toxic. All these tend to cause problem to your parts of your body with the passage of time including your thyroid gland. We become healthier once we can make use of natural items around our environments. Ensure to leave those processed foods for now. Beauty products that are toxic – free should be used. One thing that you don't know is the extent to which chemicals can damage organs and hormones in your system after some period of time.

Optimizing of Vitamin A, D as well as K2 Levels

Vitamins such as these can help promote thyroid health. They can also help your hormones function very well. It has been discovered in some studies that people who suffering from one form of thyroid disease or the other don't have much of these vitamins in their systems.

In order to obtain vitamin, spend about 30 minutes in the sunlight every day. Don't make use of sunscreen during this period since it has been discovered to block vitamin D.

Through the diet, vitamin A can be obtained. The organ meats from health animals which have been raised with pasture will be great for this.

Butter and yoke eggs are a great source of K2. Also, hard cheeses as well as kefir from cows which are healthy can also be used.

Conclusion

Once you start to implement the steps outlined you will be on the right track to heal your thyroid and feel healthier than ever before. Good luck and enjoy!

Printed in the USA
CPSIA information can be obtained
at www.ICGtesting.com
LVHW071449171223
766686LV00022B/1666